How Should Air Force Expeditionary Medical Capabilities Be Expressed?

Don Snyder, Edward W. Chan, James J. Burks,
Mahyar A. Amouzegar, Adam C. Resnick

Prepared for the United States Air Force

Approved for public release; distribution unlimited

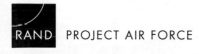

RAND PROJECT AIR FORCE

The research described in this report was sponsored by the United States Air Force under Contract FA7014-06-C-0001. Further information may be obtained from the Strategic Planning Division, Directorate of Plans, Hq USAF.

Library of Congress Cataloging-in-Publication Data

How should air force expeditionary medical capabilities be expressed? / Don Snyder ... [et al.].
     p. cm.
   Includes bibliographical references.
   ISBN 978-0-8330-4574-4 (pbk. : alk. paper)
   1. United States. Air Force—Medical care—Mathematical models.
I. Snyder, Don.

   UG983.H69 2009
   358.4'13450973—dc22

                                                                    2008054263

The RAND Corporation is a nonprofit research organization providing objective analysis and effective solutions that address the challenges facing the public and private sectors around the world. RAND's publications do not necessarily reflect the opinions of its research clients and sponsors. **RAND®** is a registered trademark.

Cover photo courtesy of U.S. Air Force/Tech. Sgt. Cecilio M. Ricardo Jr.

Published 2009 by the RAND Corporation
1776 Main Street, P.O. Box 2138, Santa Monica, CA 90407-2138
1200 South Hayes Street, Arlington, VA 22202-5050
4570 Fifth Avenue, Suite 600, Pittsburgh, PA 15213-2665
RAND URL: http://www.rand.org/
To order RAND documents or to obtain additional information, contact
Distribution Services: Telephone: (310) 451-7002;
Fax: (310) 451-6915; Email: order@rand.org

Preface

The Air Force seeks to organize and measure its expeditionary medical support in ways that are effective across the mission areas: deployed military support, humanitarian relief, and civil support. The challenge has been to find a metric of such deployed capabilities that is more suitable than the current measure, beds. The RAND Corporation was asked by the Air Force Surgeon General to devise such a metric and to develop a framework for applying it across all Air Force medical mission areas to reshape Air Force medical deployment capabilities. This monograph presents the results of that work.

The research was completed in fiscal year 2007 under a project entitled "Presenting Expeditionary Medical Capabilities." The work was sponsored by the Air Force Surgeon General and conducted within the Resource Management Program of RAND Project AIR FORCE. The monograph is intended to help the Air Force Medical Service better quantify, measure, organize, and present its ability to deploy medical support resources. It should be of interest to those working in medical planning and programming, medical logistics, modernization, and the assessment of capabilities and risks, both inside and outside the Air Force Medical Service, as well as to those involved in the mission of Defense Support to Civil Authorities.

RAND Project AIR FORCE

RAND Project AIR FORCE (PAF), a division of the RAND Corporation, is the U.S. Air Force's federally funded research and development center for studies and analyses. PAF provides the Air Force with independent analyses of policy alternatives affecting the development, employment, combat readiness, and support of current and future aerospace forces. Research is conducted in four programs: Force Modernization and Employment; Manpower, Personnel, and Training; Resource Management; and Strategy and Doctrine.

Additional information about PAF is available at
http://www.rand.org/paf/

Contents

Figures

Summary

The Air Force Medical Service (AFMS) provides care both at home stations and in deployment missions. Two platforms provide its deployment component: Expeditionary Medical Support (EMEDS) and the aeromedical evacuation system. These have evolved over the years to provide increasingly better care to service members during deployments. Much of this success can be credited to the concept of operations (CONOPS) of these systems and the tailoring of manpower and equipment to that concept.

The operational emphasis of expeditionary medicine is on patient flow. An injured patient receives limited treatment locally and is then moved from the point of injury to an EMEDS facility as quickly as possible. There, the patient is further evaluated, stabilized, triaged, treated, and evacuated to a higher level of care. Each level of care is designed to be sufficient for immediate needs, not to provide definitive care. This emphasis on flow streamlines capabilities that need to be deployed and places the definitive care in the most capable facilities. Although this framework has functioned well for the mission of supporting the warfighter, two areas need improvement.

First, the most common current measure of capability, both within but especially outside the Air Force, is the number of available "beds." Yet, other than the final inpatient facilities that provide definitive care, the components of the expeditionary en route medical system are not intended to hold patients per se. Rather, patients are processed as quickly as is prudent and handed off to the next level to receive further care. The measure of beds does not adequately reflect this concept of operations, and requests that are stated in terms of beds are not likely to deliver the proper set of resources to meet the real requirements.

Second, EMEDS is designed to provide the needed capabilities in warfighting missions, which consist predominantly of providing trauma care to relatively young and otherwise healthy patients. However, in humanitarian relief missions and the provision of defense support to civil authorities, fewer trauma patients present. Patients range from children to the elderly, with men and women represented similarly, and many of them have chronic medical or psychiatric conditions. Sending EMEDS to meet these needs often deploys trauma and surgical capabilities that are not needed and fails to furnish the required supplies and the personnel with the appropriate range of skills to care for the full scope of patient conditions.

Both of these deficiencies can be improved with a fresh perspective on the capability metric for medical deployments. A capability metric that captures the dynamic aspects of the en route expeditionary medical mission rather than a static measure of beds can enable the right resources to be placed to meet the requirements of the full range of medical deployments.

In this study, we focused on the throughput of patients, defining a metric of capability for the *rate* at which each component of the deployment system can stabilize, triage and treat, and evacuate patients, or the *medical STEP rate*. The acronym captures the quality of flow through a system and implies that each element of the system provides an important step within it. Our concept involves determining the medical STEP rate required for deployments and building unit type codes (UTCs) to meet those STEP rates. The UTCs could be highly modular and able to be assembled rapidly to meet a wide range of needed capabilities without either deploying significant unneeded capabilities or highly tailoring the UTCs.

Medical STEP rates can be estimated in advance during deliberate planning for the mission to support the warfighter. However, predicting in advance is problematic for the humanitarian relief and defense support to civil authorities missions. Nevertheless, the metric captures more closely the requirement at the time of need than does the measure of the number of beds. Because of the aptness of the metric, it could be used by medical planners and logisticians to recommend and request appropriate forces to meet needs during crisis action planning.

For a component such as EMEDS, the resources needed to achieve a desired medical STEP rate for a given patient condition type will depend largely on two factors of a deployment: the conditions of the patients and the rates at which patients arrive and are able to move to the next, higher level of care. We propose first defining a limited number of patient condition types. Then, UTCs could potentially be created that enable patients of a given type to be accepted at a certain medical STEP rate. Since it would be impractical to create UTCs for every patient condition, patient conditions might be grouped into a small, manageable number of types. Further research could shed more light on the choices, but one possibility would be to adopt the standard categories used in triage during any mass-casualty situation. The categories, in decreasing order of priority, are *urgent, immediate, delayed, minimal,* and *deceased* (or expectant).[1]

Patients will arrive in one of these categories at some rate that may vary over time. For each condition type, resources would be assembled into UTCs to achieve a given STEP rate. Achieving higher medical STEP rates would be accomplished by using additional UTCs of the same types. The rate at which patients arrive will not affect the *types* of resources needed, as these are determined by the patient conditions. However, the rates of arrival and outflow will affect the medical STEP rate needed. Patients with various conditions will require different levels of resources, different types of supplies and equipment, and different manpower skills. Also, the rate at which the receiving components of the en route system can accept the patients from a deployed facility will affect the holding capacity that facility needs.

If UTCs or combinations of modular UTCs existed for several medical STEP rates for each of the classical triage categories, defense coordinating officers would have an adequate vocabulary with which to relay the needs, and the Air Force could have the appropriate resources ready to meet those needs. This modularity would also facilitate the

---

[1] Craig H. Llewellyn, "Triage: In Austere Environments and Echeloned Medical Systems," *World Journal of Surgery,* Vol. 16, 1992, pp. 904–909.

deployment of capabilities matched to the deployment needs without significant tailoring of UTCs, thereby increasing the speed at which capabilities can be deployed and reducing the delivery of unneeded resources. The use of a medical STEP rate rather than available beds as the capability metric seems to hold the promise of providing a more agile, responsive, and effective medical deployment capability.

Acknowledgments

This work was sponsored by the Air Force Deputy Surgeon General, Maj Gen C. Bruce Green, and could not have been done without his advice and support. We had numerous discussions during which we learned about the issues surrounding medical deployments and how military support situations differ from those encountered in civil support and humanitarian relief. Among the many people who participated in these discussions, we especially thank Maj Gen Thomas Loftus, Brig Gen Theresa Casey, Col Richard Hersack, Col Cheryl Gregorio, Col Randall Hagan, Col Ivan Sherard, Col Rudolph Cachuela, Col Linda Ebling, CAPT Jeff Timby, Lt Col Linda Cashion, Lt Col Corie Culver, Lt Col Nancy Klein, Maj Ed LaGrou, Capt Joe Lyons, and Lew Rissmiller (ranks are those at the time of our meetings).

Col Robert Bowersox and Maj Mike Foutch served as excellent action officers throughout the project.

At RAND, we benefited from numerous discussions and feedback. In particular, we thank Laura Baldwin, Maj Andrew Baxter, David Johnson, Edward Keating, Melinda Moore, and C. Robert Roll, Jr. Gary Cecchine and Tom LaTourrette provided us with constructive reviews that substantially improved this monograph, but we alone are responsible for any errors or oversights that may remain.

Abbreviations

AEF	Aerospace Expeditionary Force
AFMS	Air Force Medical Service
AFTH	Air Force Theater Hospital
AMC	Air Mobility Command
ATH	air transportable hospital
CASEVAC	casualty evacuation
CASF	Contingency Aeromedical Staging Facility
CCATT	Critical Care Air Transport Team
CONOPS	concept of operations
DMAT	Disaster Medical Assistance Team
DNBI	disease and non-battle injury
DoD	Department of Defense
DSCA	Defense Support to Civil Authorities
EMEDS	Expeditionary Medical Support
ESF	Emergency Support Function
HUMRO	humanitarian relief operation
ICU	intensive care unit
MASF	Mobile Aeromedical Staging Facility
MEDEVAC	medical evacuation

NDMS   National Disaster Medical System

PAR   population at risk

SPEARR   Small Portable Expeditionary Aeromedical Rapid Response

STEP   stabilize, triage and treat, and evacuate patients

TACC   Tanker Airlift Control Center

TAES   Theater Aeromedical Evacuation System

TTTF   Task, Time, Treater File

UTC   unit type code

CHAPTER ONE

Introduction

Modern technological advances have furnished new and more deadly ways to inflict injury during battle. But modern technological advances have also provided the Air Force Medical Service (AFMS) with the means to prevent more service personnel dying from non-battle diseases and to enable more service personnel to survive battle and non-battle injuries.[1] Many changes—including technological advances, better organization, and improved processes—have led to this improvement of military medical care.

One set of evolutionary changes that has increased survival rates comprises advancements in the way medical capabilities are deployed and employed. In particular, the development of expeditionary medical treatment facilities and aeromedical evacuation has greatly reduced the time between injury and receiving the appropriate level of medical care.[2] These modern improvements began back in the Korean War, and the concepts continue to evolve.[3]

The first modern medical deployment facilities resulted from the creation and evolution of the air transportable hospital (ATH) and its

---

[1] Richard A. Gabriel and Karen S. Metz, *A History of Military Medicine, Volume 2: From the Renaissance Through Modern Times*, New York: Greenwood Press, 1992; John T. Greenwood and F. Clifton Berry, Jr., *Medics at War: Military Medicine from Colonial Times to the 21st Century*, Annapolis, Md.: Naval Institute Press, 2005.

[2] Five levels of care are defined, ranging from the unit level up to definitive care at a facility such as a major hospital. See the Appendix in *Health Services*, Air Force Doctrine Document 2-4.2, 11 December 2002.

[3] Office the Air Force Surgeon General, n.d.

associated concept of operations (CONOPS),[4] the goal of which was to provide a robust in-theater treatment and holding facility. Deployed ATHs had 14, 25, or 50 beds, with the latter supporting up to 4,000 patients. The 50-bed version required six C-141 cargo planes for movement.[5]

As evidenced by the large number of beds, the ATH facilities emphasized care in place (in theater) rather than being individual components in a medical network that prepared patients for movement to higher levels of care. In 1998, concurrent with the development of the Aerospace Expeditionary Force (AEF) construct, the AFMS began refashioning deployable medical capabilities into a new structure called Expeditionary Medical Support (EMEDS), the goal of which was to reduce the theater footprint and decrease the time to deployment and employment. First deployed in 1999 in support of Operation Allied Force in the Balkans, EMEDS is still used by the Air Force to organize and deploy its medical capabilities.

We will describe and discuss EMEDS in more detail below, but briefly, it is a modular, scalable set of deployable medical equipment and manpower. It dovetails with the aeromedical evacuation system to provide rapid treatment and movement of patients to higher levels of care. The EMEDS capability is measured by the number of medical "beds" that it can provide. The basic form of EMEDS can be augmented by 10 beds or 25 beds with an "EMEDS + 10" or "EMEDS + 25" supplementation.

During deployments, the CONOPS is to move patients, via the aeromedical evacuation system, through increasing levels of medical care, of which the EMEDS deployable facility is just one step, albeit a central one. This reduces the deployment footprint of the facility and defers higher levels of care to more-capable, definitive care facilities,

---

[4] Peter Dorland and James S. Nanney, *Dust Off: Army Aeromedical Evacuation in Vietnam*, Washington, D.C.: Center of Military History, United States Army, 1982.

[5] James S. Nanney, *The Air Force Medical Service in the Persian Gulf War*, Bolling AFB, Washington, D.C.: United States Air Force, Office of the Surgeon General, 1992; James S. Nanney, *The Air Force Medical Service and the Persian Gulf War: A Ten-Year Retrospective*, Bolling AFB, Washington, D.C.: United States Air Force, Office of the Surgeon General, n.d.

usually outside the theater of operations. The lessons learned from the Korean War onward have produced EMEDS capabilities and CONOPS that are highly evolved and integrated with the medical evacuation system. Nevertheless, two areas remain for improvement.

First, EMEDS is designed specifically for the expeditionary warfighting mission, i.e., to support military personnel deployed at locations supported by the Air Force. Although EMEDS has served this role well, it supports humanitarian relief operations (HUMROs) and Defense Support to Civil Authorities (DSCA) missions somewhat awkwardly. EMEDS has a surgical focus and provides manpower and supplies catered to the mission of caring for traumatic injuries to a relatively young, otherwise healthy population. In contrast, patients encountered in the HUMRO and DSCA missions present, in general, proportionately fewer trauma injuries, and the overall population contains more children, elderly, and chronically ill patients. The balance of capabilities in EMEDS currently does not meet the full spectrum of these needs.

Second, and more fundamentally, the measure of "beds" does not satisfactorily reflect the capability that EMEDS provides: a key, deployable element of a medical network that moves patients as needed up through higher levels of medical care. The number of beds merely reflects some measure of the holding capacity of a facility. It does not reflect the ability of the facility to evaluate, stabilize, triage, treat, and prepare patients with differing conditions for transport to higher levels of care. A better measure is needed, both to articulate the capability to requesters and to better shape EMEDS resources to meet the needs expressed by this new measure.

A plea regarding EMEDS made after Hurricane Katrina by then Air Force Surgeon General Lt Gen (Dr) George Taylor, Jr., captures both issues:

> What we are grappling with is finding the basic measure of medical capabilities in this new world of rapid transportation. In the past, we've used the term "bed" as the basic building block for the medics. But in an era when we have the capability to move large numbers of patients quickly and effectively to higher levels

of care, isn't the flow from a location at least as important as the beds there? . . . In the case of Hurricane Katrina, the Air Force moved thousands of patients from New Orleans to hospitals in Dallas, San Antonio, Atlanta and Houston without a large, formal bedded facility.[6]

In response to this call for a more suitable metric of capability and the desire to meet the needs of the HUMRO and DSCA missions more flexibly and precisely, this study posits and explores an alternative measure of deployable medical capabilities and discusses how capabilities might be organized and measured employing it.

This new measure embraces the concepts of patient flow through the various elements of the deployed medical network, focusing on EMEDS, and abandons the static measure of beds. We will outline how such a measure might be used to determine the resources needed to optimize patient flow and how those resources might be assembled to provide the requisite EMEDS capabilities. We argue that changing perspective from beds to a measure that emphasizes patient flow can also help meet the full spectrum of mission needs. We further argue that adopting this measure and organizing forces according to it can mitigate many of the deficiencies in the current medical support for the HUMRO and DSCA missions. Further work will be required to determine what flow rates should be supported and what resources are required to meet these rates, but this monograph develops the overall conceptual frame for doing so.

Chapter Two examines the three expeditionary medical missions, highlighting the role of deployable medical resources. Chapter Three briefly examines the limitations of these current processes and resources, then outlines a new paradigm for expeditionary medical deployment that revolves around the new capability measure. Chapter Four provides a brief summary of the study. The Appendix reviews how expeditionary medical treatment is currently organized and provides a more detailed description of both EMEDS and aeromedical evacuation.

---

[6] G. W. Pomeroy, "Dividends from OEF, OIF Pay Off for Medics in Katrina Aftermath," *Air Force Print News Today*, 30 September 2005.

CHAPTER TWO

Air Force Medical Deployment Missions

The AFMS is called upon to provide deployable medical care to support deployed military personnel (i.e., the warfighting mission), to provide care to residents in other countries during HUMRO, and to support other government agencies in providing medical assistance to U.S. residents during disasters at home (i.e., the DSCA mission). Currently, the Air Force can plan and program for only two of these missions: warfighting and HUMRO.

The Air Force is not the lead agency for medical assistance for the DSCA mission, but it nonetheless can fashion robust capabilities for warfighting and HUMRO in such a way that they also serve effectively and seamlessly in DSCA. Each of these missions presents different challenges for the AFMS. To organize and shape expeditionary medical capabilities to meet all three missions, we must first understand the attributes they have in common and the unique demands that each presents.

How can the AFMS better adapt to these disparate mission environments? For this, we need to understand in more detail the individual demands of the deployment missions the AFMS fulfills. In this chapter, we examine the characteristics of these mission areas that any deployable medical capability must meet. These common elements then serve as a guide for formulating a new measure of capability. Throughout, we assume familiarity with the current deployed Air Force medical capabilities and CONOPS. The current state is summarized in the Appendix.

For all three missions, we focus on how the deployable facility is situated within its surrounding environment during deployments. Along with the nature of the conditions of the presenting patients, which we take up later, two important characteristics are the nature of the influx of patients to the deployed facility and the nature of the outflow of patients from it. Figure 2.1 illustrates this surrounding environment schematically.

On the influx side, patients arrive at the facility at a given rate that may be difficult to predict in advance. It may be fairly constant over time, or it may vary considerably. Superimposed on this arrival distribution are the conditions of the patients who present, which range from having no problems requiring medical care to requiring urgent treatment. The conditions of the patients and the rate of arrival may or may not be correlated. Both the distribution of patient arrival rates and

Figure 2.1
Environment Surrounding a Deployed Medical Facility

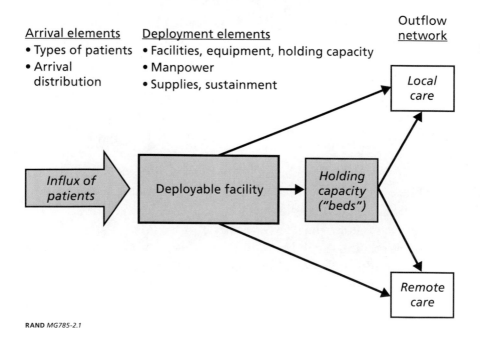

RAND MG785-2.1

the nature of conditions differ across and, to a lesser degree, within the three missions.

On the outflow side, the key relationship is the operation of the deployable capability as part of a larger medical network. Rarely does such a deployed facility operate in isolation, exclusively providing definitive care and never moving patients to another medical facility. More commonly, it functions as part of a medical network, much as a clinic or some hospitals do in the United States. It is not intended to be a definitive care facility. Rather, its function is to evaluate patients, perform triage, treat, and stabilize them enough to enable them to be transferred to a higher level of care.

That higher level of care may be present locally or may be at some distance. If the deployable capability is meant to supplement other locally available capabilities, as it might be during a DSCA mission, it may be set up outside or near a major hospital, medical shelter, or palliative care unit. In these situations, patient transfer may be simple, involving no more than ambulances. If the deployable capability is quite remote from the available higher levels of care, as it might be during the warfighting mission, a more sophisticated aeromedical evacuation system may be required.

Two factors determine the need for a holding capacity at a deployed facility: (1) whether the patients, once treated, need to recover before moving on to the next step in the treatment process (or being released), and (2) when the outflow system cannot handle the rate at which the deployed facility is prepared to release patients. This mismatch in rates causes a buildup of patients, which requires a holding capacity. We return to this concept later when we discuss setting the appropriate level of medical resources to meet mission needs.

The key to structuring robust deployable medical capabilities is to define and quantify—across the three mission areas—the aspects these environments have in common and the aspects that differ. In the following sections, we describe the mission areas, emphasizing salient aspects of the deployment environment: patient influx and outflow. These observations will form the fabric for fashioning robust and transparently understandable deployable medical capabilities and capacities for the deployable medical facility. This will serve as the basis for future quantification of medical deployment requirements.

The Mission to Support the Warfighter

In the usual setting for which Air Force expeditionary medical support was designed, i.e., supporting expeditionary combat operations, most of the patients are military service personnel. They tend to be young and in generally good health, as they will have been considered healthy enough to deploy. The primary reason for seeking medical attention will be trauma injuries, from both routine military operations and the battlefield.

The Air Force estimates that in wartime settings, some 80 percent of patients present with disease and non-battle injuries (DNBI).[1] These patients are not likely to be suffering from chronic medical conditions. Wartime operations may also result in civilian casualties. While these casualties are trauma patients, they represent a wider demographic range than that of military personnel. Patient arrivals due to DNBI are fairly steady, punctuated by intervals of higher arrivals, such as during infectious-disease outbreaks.

Patients suffering battlefield injuries may arrive singly or in batches, depending on the size of the incident and the means by which patients are transported to the treatment facility, e.g., by casualty evacuation (CASEVAC). In addition, the day-to-day or week-to-week rate of patients may differ, depending on the operations tempo of combat activities.

The expeditionary treatment facility, while capable, is still an austere facility in comparison to a major hospital and is limited in size and resources. In an expeditionary wartime setting, local fixed facility hospitals are likely to be unavailable or undesirable except as options of last resort. The expeditionary treatment facility itself, while removed from

---

[1] *Expeditionary Medical Support (EMEDS)*, Air Force Tactics, Techniques, and Procedures 3-42.71, 27 July 2006, section 1.3.2.1.

the battlefield, may yet be in an area subject to attack. Consequently, the CONOPS in treating wartime casualties is to evacuate them out of the theater as soon as they are stabilized enough to be transported, so that they can receive higher levels of care out of harm's way in Europe or the United States.

We can summarize this concept by a generalized example (details will vary according to circumstances). When a service member is injured in the battlefield, he or she receives in the field the immediate care that can be provided by comrades in order to stabilize him or her for transport to an expeditionary treatment facility provided by EMEDS. At the EMEDS unit, a higher level of care is available. The patient is further evaluated and treated, possibly undergoing surgery.

In some cases, the patient may be released following treatment at the EMEDS facility after being held and observed for some time. In general, however, the EMEDS is not intended to provide definitive care, i.e., completion of all recommended treatment, even when surgery is performed. The goal is to provide the care needed to prepare the patient for transport out of the theater to a major medical hospital. In current operations in Iraq, injured service personnel are typically transported to the Landstuhl Regional Medical Center, Germany. Treatment resumes there, and the patients may be further transferred to a rehabilitation center in the United States.

The operational emphasis is on patient flow. Each step—stabilization and any treatment in the field, EMEDS, a major hospital, and rehabilitation—provides what is needed at that juncture, deferring higher-level treatment to the next step in the flow. The deployable components (i.e., EMEDS) can thus be leaner and deployed and redeployed more rapidly, and the patient can receive definitive treatment in a higher-level facility. In contrast to the ATH described in Chapter One, the system is streamlined and agile, and the deployment timelines are reduced.

The HUMRO Mission

Air Force doctrine describes foreign HUMROs as an "umbrella term" that includes missions undertaken to alleviate human suffering, disease, or hunger that result from natural or man-made disasters.[2] These operations may be the primary mission (e.g., response to the Southeast Asia tsunami and the earthquake in Pakistan), or they may be secondary to ongoing military operations. HUMROs can also be conducted under the auspices of training in support of a combatant-commander-directed preplanned mission (e.g., a medical-readiness training exercise to provide medical care in underdeveloped nations under the theater-commander engagement strategies). In the case of disasters, the impact of the event determines the duration for which relief is necessary. In general, the U.S. military does not maintain a long-term presence in the affected area after the initial response, transitioning responsibilities for longer-term assistance to domestic and international governmental and non-governmental organizations (for instance, the U.S. Department of State/U.S. Agency for International Development or the International Red Cross).

Not all HUMRO activities look alike. They vary, depending on a number of contextual factors. Responding organizations—governmental and non-governmental organizations from the United States and the international community—encounter a range of logistical demands, including finding serviceable airfields, lack of infrastructure, and lack of host-nation capabilities to assist in the response. These contextual factors influence the nature of the patient influx into a deployable medical facility and the outflow from that facility. Existing medical facilities may also be damaged or overwhelmed by the disaster, but this plays a smaller role in HUMRO planning than it does in the DSCA mission, as the HUMRO response generally operates autonomously of any indigenous medical facilities.

In contrast to the warfighting mission, the patients that present in the HUMRO mission are not predominantly young and fit, and the most common medical condition may not be trauma. Those needing medical attention may have suffered injuries due to a disaster, or

---

[2] *Health Services*, Air Force Doctrine Document 2-4.2, 11 December 2002.

they may need care because their local facilities have been damaged or are inadequate. Also, the emergency responders themselves may need medical care. Hence, the patients in a HUMRO typically represent a much wider sample of the general population, ranging from children to the elderly, and they may have chronic medical conditions or mental health problems.

The rate of patients' arrival may also differ significantly from that in the warfighting mission. In the warfighting mission, the medical capabilities will ideally be deployed and employed before significant patient arrival. In the HUMRO mission, however, a large queue of patients may have already formed prior to the arrival of the expeditionary medical capability because of a catastrophic disaster or because medical care has been inadequate in the region for some time. Hence, a large number of patients may present, placing a severe burden on triage and the need for a large initial capacity to treat patients.

The DSCA Mission

The DSCA mission, as distinct from HUMRO missions, is the Department of Defense (DoD) provision of disaster relief in the United States and its territories. The lead for the various relief roles is divided among the federal departments, with non-lead departments serving a supporting role. The lead falls to the Department of Health and Human Services for medical assistance during federal relief in domestic disasters; DoD acts in a supporting role according to Emergency Support Function (ESF) #8.[3] Much has been learned from the experience in the aftermath of Hurricane Katrina, but it is imperative to keep in mind that the Katrina experience may not be typical of future incidents and should not be viewed as an exemplar for all disaster relief.[4] Disasters

---

[3] *National Response Framework*, Washington, D.C.: Department of Homeland Security, January 2008.

[4] T. Michael Moseley, *Air Force Support to Hurricane Katrina/Rita Relief Operations: Successes and Challenges*, Washington D.C.: Office of the Chief of Staff of the U.S. Air Force, August–September 2005; Crystal Franco, Eric Toner, Richard Waldhorn, Beth Maldin, Tara O'Toole, and Thomas V. Inglesby, "Systemic Collapse: Medical Care in the Aftermath

range from the expected, such as hurricanes and earthquakes, to less frequent but consequential events such as volcanic eruptions and terrorist attacks involving weapons of mass destruction.

Air Force doctrine[5] recognizes that a major disaster or emergency will cause numerous fatalities and injuries, property loss, and disruption of normal life-support systems and will almost always have an impact on a region's economic, physical, and social infrastructures. The extent of a disaster's impact is determined by factors such as weather conditions, population density, infrastructure, and secondary events such as fires, floods, and domestic unrest (i.e., looting and lawlessness). Civilian medical facilities—including inpatient hospitals, outpatient care centers, and local pharmacies—may be damaged, destroyed, or rendered unusable due to the disaster's impact on utilities or staff members' abilities to physically respond. Medical facilities that are operational may be overwhelmed by patients, ranging from those with true emergent conditions (life-, limb-, or eyesight-threatening), to the "walking wounded," to the "walking worried." Medical supplies and equipment may be in short supply.

Additionally, uninjured persons who require daily or frequent medications or treatments (e.g., insulin, antihypertensive drugs, chemotherapy, dialysis) may not be able to access these supplies or services, causing health effects ranging from deleterious to deadly. Public health and bioenvironmental issues (e.g., disease vectors and damage to water supplies, respectively) may also result from a disaster. Finally, some events—including an attack using weapons of mass destruction—could overwhelm federal, state, and local public health and medical care capabilities.

Like the patients served in the HUMRO mission, patients in domestic disaster situations will be civilians and first responders of all

---

of Hurricane Katrina," *Biosecurity and Bioterrorism: Biodefense Strategy, Practice, and Science*, Vol. 4, 2006, pp. 135–146; Sarah A. Lister, *Hurricane Katrina: The Public Health and Medical Response*, CRS Report for Congress, Washington, D.C.: Congressional Research Service, 21 September 2005; Steve Bowman, Lawrence Kapp, and Amy Belasco, *Hurricane Katrina: DoD Disaster Response*, CRS Report for Congress, Washington, D.C.: Congressional Research Service, 19 September 2005.

[5] *Health Services*, Air Force Doctrine Document 2-4.2, 2002.

ages with a variety of underlying medical conditions. The vast majority of patients who were victims of Hurricane Katrina required care for existing chronic medical conditions, such as diabetes, high blood pressure, and mental health issues, problems that were exacerbated by the loss of access to their usual health care providers resulting from damage to the infrastructure.[6]

One possible reason for expeditionary treatment facilities used in disaster response situations not seeing many patients suffering from trauma is the timing of the arrival of the facilities. Whereas in wartime, facilities are set up and receive new casualties produced over the course of the war, in a disaster situation, the bulk of the injuries are often produced at once, and the responding treatment facility arrives later.

By the time the facility is set up, patients with injuries requiring immediate care either will have already been cared for or will have died. The large number of patients awaiting the arrival of the medical care facility will likely be those previously triaged as "delayed" or "minor" whose care has been deferred because existing medical facilities are damaged or overwhelmed. The goal of the expeditionary facility is to provide care to these patients so that their injuries or chronic conditions do not become acute conditions or immediate threats to life or limb.

The goal in wartime settings is to evacuate patients from the theater, but in domestic disaster situations, evacuation may not be as desirable, as this removes patients from their home area. Interviews with local emergency medical officials and federal civilian disaster medical responders indicate a desire to not "export the disaster." The role of the expeditionary medical facility, then, is less as a gateway to evacuation and more as a filter on the flow of patients to the available nearby fixed treatment facilities. Evacuation out of the area may still be needed, however, if there is widespread infrastructure damage that renders existing fixed treatment facilities unavailable or if the number of casualties overwhelms the available capacity in local hospitals.

---

[6] Based on discussions with first responders from the U.S. Northern Command (NORTHCOM) and Disaster Medical Assistance Teams (DMAT).

Comparing and Contrasting the HUMRO and DSCA Missions

There are many parallels in the HUMRO and DSCA environments. Patient influx in both presents a full range of demographics and chronic conditions, unlike the mission to support the warfighter, where the demographics are more restricted and trauma is more expected. However, there are some important distinctions between them.

First, although in both situations infrastructure damage may limit or overwhelm the local medical facilities, the consequences for the Air Force deploying forces differ. In many HUMRO cases, the United States operates nearly autonomously of host-nation facilities, which simplifies planning and operations. That is not to say that the U.S. military does not cooperate with host nations, but it need not integrate its operations into those of the host nation and can exercise full command and control of its assets and medical evacuation system. In the DSCA mission, the situation is more complicated. Here, the military is a supporting element and must work within the National Response Framework, which may mean integrating within the capabilities of the existing infrastructure.

Second, the Air Force can set requirements, organize its forces, and program its capabilities to support HUMROs, while the DSCA mission is not within its programming purview. This difference makes highlighting the similarities that do exist between the two missions important. In areas in which the demands of the mission coincide, changes made for the HUMRO mission can also facilitate the DSCA mission. This supports the DSCA role without explicitly dedicating any resources to it. In the next chapter, we discuss the issue of how well the current materiel and CONOPS serve the three mission areas.

CHAPTER THREE

A New Concept for Air Force Medical Deployment Capabilities

In this chapter, we first review some of the limitations of the current expeditionary medical capabilities in the three missions. We then draw some generalizations across these areas and use them to motivate a fresh look at how deployable medical capabilities should be fashioned and their capabilities measured. The keystone to defining and measuring capabilities will be a new metric, which is the focus of the latter half of the chapter.

General Characteristics of the Mission Areas

Supporting the Warfighter

EMEDS and aeromedical evacuation are designed specifically for the mission to support the warfighter. We are unaware of any chronic problems with EMEDS for this mission that affect the metrics discussed here.

The HUMRO and DSCA Missions

As stated earlier, HUMRO and DSCA have distinct requirements, although a response package tailored for the former may be appropriate for the latter. For both missions, current Air Force-deployable assets may not be modularized in a manner that best fits civil disaster response. A civil disaster that significantly damages or destroys civilian health-care infrastructure requires a community-medicine-based response, which is different from a medical response to a combat scenario. Also, the populations at risk and the patients' needs differ. Similarities and differences between the two missions' requirements are discussed below.

Several lessons observed from the Hurricane Katrina response inform this discussion.[1] The first is recognition of a significant limiting factor in a post-disaster scenario: the timeline for an immediate life-saving response, especially if civil medical capabilities are rendered largely inoperable. One could reasonably expect a lag in response time from state and federal authorities based on factors such as post-incident "all-clear"/safety considerations, distance to and location of disaster, mobilization time, coordination requirements, logistics requirements (movement of supplies and equipment), and infrastructure status (destroyed roads and/or bridges). The planning factor for the arrival of Title X forces is approximately 96 hours.[2]

Once a medical capability is in place, patient-holding capacity (i.e., beds) is not necessarily what is required in the immediate post-incident period (the first 72 hours). The response to Hurricane Katrina demonstrated the compelling need to triage patients, stabilize those in immediate medical distress, and release or transfer them quickly and appropriately. Furthermore, during that response, it was observed that medication requirements for a civil response differ greatly from those in a combat scenario (for instance, the need for insulin).

The scope of services provided by military assets under various scenarios and the implications of the decision to provide services must be determined in advance by disaster planners. Military responders could be asked to care for the population as a whole or could be asked to provide care only to responding forces and agencies. This decision has

---

[1] Frances Fragos Townsend, *The Federal Response to Hurricane Katrina: Lessons Learned*, Washington D.C.: The White House, February 2006; Lynn E. Davis, Jill Rough, Gary Cecchine, Agnes Gereben Schaefer, and Laurinda L. Zeman, *Hurricane Katrina: Lessons for Army Planning and Operations*, Santa Monica, Calif.: RAND Corporation, MG-603-A, 2007; William B. Scott, David A. Fulghum, and Craig Covault, "The Second Storm," *Aviation Week and Space Technology*, 12 September 2005, pp. 20–22.; Franco et al., 2006.

[2] Gary Cecchine, RAND Corporation, personal communication, March 2008.

great implications for the way a capability is tailored for a post-disaster response, such as the personnel and resources that will be provided.

Common Environmental Elements Across Air Force Medical Missions

To build a new measure of deployed medical capabilities, we first look at the patient flow at a forward expeditionary medical treatment facility and describe it in general terms that apply to the support of the warfighter, HUMRO, and DSCA missions.

Patient Influx

We characterize the inputs to the medical facility—i.e., the patients— in three areas: type of injury or illness of patients, severity of patient conditions, and arrival pattern of patients.

We first group patients on the basis of their chief complaint. They may be trauma patients, with injuries or wounds caused by external force, including battle injuries or accidents, or they may present with conditions caused by disease or other internal conditions. These conditions may be acute (rapid onset) or chronic (long-term, progressing gradually). Categorization of patients as trauma or medical is useful for determining the type of care they will require.

Next, we categorize patients by the severity of their conditions, which is more important for the purpose of measuring flow and throughput. We use the standard categories used in triage during any mass-casualty situation where the number of patients threatens to overwhelm the number of caregivers. The categories, in decreasing order of priority, are *urgent, immediate, delayed, minimal,* and *deceased* (or expectant).[3] The categorization is useful for determining the order in which patients will be treated, regardless of the underlying causes of their ailments. Also, categorizing patients by severity can provide an indication of the personnel and time that will be spent caring for them, as patients with more severe conditions will presumably require more

---

[3] Llewellyn, 1992.

resources than those with less severe conditions, at least when it comes to emergency care.

Finally, we consider the arrival pattern of the patients, which is associated less with individual patients than with the overall flow. Patients arrive at a medical facility by their own power or are brought by first responders such as buddies, medics, or some form of casualty evacuation (CASEVAC). They may trickle in, in small numbers in a more-or-less random pattern over time, the way they might in a normal, everyday environment with disease and non-battle injuries (DNBI). Alternatively, they may arrive in large batches, as would be expected in a multiple-casualty accident, an outbreak, or CASEVAC from the battlefield. The number of patients arriving at any one time affects the ability of the facility to treat each of them, as well as the level of care that may be provided, and is one of the factors governing the number of patients held at the facility.

Patient Outflow

In Figure 2.1 of Chapter Two, we outlined broad categories of patient outflow (i.e., the various ways in which patients leave an expeditionary medical facility): patients held at the deployed facility, patients moved to another local facility, and patients moved to a remote facility (e.g., via aeromedical evacuation). In this section, we discuss these possibilities in more detail, and for completeness we add the possibility that patients are treated and released. The important issue in all these cases will be how rapidly the outflow network can receive patients, not the details of what the downstream components of the network might look like in terms of care. We do discuss some possibilities regarding types of care, however, in order to draw attention to the ways rates of accepting patients downstream of a deployed facility might vary.

Treat and Release the Patient. The patient may be held at the facility for a brief period of observation after treatment, but there is no overnight stay. There is no limitation on the ability of the deployed facility to receive patients if they are released after treatment.

Hold the Patient at the Deployed Facility. Patients may require further treatment at the level of care provided by the treatment facility. Such treatment may include surgery and hospitalization. While appropriate for a civilian fixed facility (i.e., a hospital) in normal operations, holding patients for further treatment is not a preferred course of action for expeditionary medical treatment facilities because of the limited space and resources available, as described above. Nevertheless, the facility must have holding capacity sufficient to meet the admission needs.

Treat and Transfer the Patient to a Local Facility. We distinguish three cases in which patients are treated and transferred. First the patient may be transferred to a facility that provides a *lower* level of care. In this case, the patient does not require hospitalization but requires some continued care and should not simply be released unattended. In a normal health-care setting this might mean releasing the patient to a nursing home. In a domestic civilian disaster setting, it may mean releasing the patient to some form of medical shelter, such as a Red Cross shelter or a Federal Medical Station staffed by the U.S. Public Health Service or DMAT. The medical treatment facility itself might need to hold the patient while awaiting transport or evacuation.

Second, the patient may be transferred to a facility that provides a higher level of care. This would be necessary if the receiving facility lacks the capacity or capability to handle the patient. Just about any fixed hospital (short of those in developing nations) would be considered a more advanced facility than an expeditionary medical treatment facility, and consequently this course of action could be taken in a domestic disaster-response situation if hospitals with sufficient capacity and capability are available nearby. Patients may also be transferred from a fixed-facility civilian hospital to more advanced trauma, brain injury, or burn centers within the area. For our purposes, we consider nearby facilities to be those reachable by ground ambulance or, at most, rotary-winged aircraft.

Third, patients may be transferred to a palliative care facility. Patients who are expectant, for whom the decision has been made that no further definitive care will be given, may be transferred to a setting where palliative care may be provided to give comfort and ease pain.

The decision of whether and where to transfer patients will depend on the severity of their conditions, the capability and capacity at the receiving facility, and the supporting medical and transportation infrastructure available.

Treat and Transfer the Patient to a Remote Facility. Here we distinguish among the mission areas. Most commonly, patients who are moved outside the theater of activity during the warfighting mission are transferred to a facility that provides a higher level of care. That facility is likely to be an established institution and will be expecting to receive patients. In the DSCA mission, patients may be moved to a higher or lower level of care, depending on the circumstances. In either case, the arrangements are likely to be ad hoc. We are unaware of any plans to transport patients in HUMRO operations to remote facilities. In all cases, the availability of mobility forces to move the patients and the limited capability of receiving facilities might require a holding capacity at the deployed medical facility.

A New Paradigm for Deployable Medical Capabilities

Several common themes recur in the above description and discussion of the expeditionary portion of the AFMS mission. These hold regardless of the type of mission. The most important attribute is that the deployable capability, EMEDS, does not function as an isolated element. It serves as a component in a system that provides medical care via an agile, coordinated network of two interleaved capabilities. The first capability provides medical care at various levels ranging from Small Portable Expeditionary Aeromedical Rapid Response (SPEARR) teams to definitive-care hospitals. The second capability provides medically supervised transport among these locations and facilities. Adequate measures of performance of components in this system must reflect their interdependence and how they contribute to the overall care of a patient as he or she flows through the network.

Observations on the Legacy Measure: Beds

The most common current measure of capability is the number of beds in a facility. The required level of beds is driven by the population at risk (PAR). Beds are a convenient unit of measure: They are readily observed, easily counted, and thus easily quantified. Fixed-facility hospitals describe their capacity in terms of beds, and civilian government emergency-services agencies and health departments likewise track the number of beds available among the hospitals in their region.

Even as the Air Force has promoted the notion that EMEDS provides only forward medical intervention and must be complemented by timely aeromedical evacuation of casualties, it has continued to categorize its EMEDS configurations in terms of the number of inpatient beds each possesses, e.g., EMEDS + 10 and EMEDS + 25. The unfortunate implication is that the number of beds corresponds to the number of patients who can be treated.

Measuring the capability of expeditionary medical support in terms of beds is misleading because making a one-to-one correspondence between the number of beds in a facility and the total number of patients who can be cared for implicitly assumes that patients will be occupying beds for an extended period of time. It puts the focus on inpatient care, where patients spend an extended amount of time undergoing definitive care that may include further treatment, surgery, and recovery. It assumes that inpatient care is provided at the expeditionary facility and that the patient is retained until he or she has recovered.

But this notion is contrary to the CONOPS for expeditionary medical support described earlier. Today, the AFMS thinks of its continuum of medical capabilities in terms of the "en route system"—i.e., the Air Force contributions to the joint patient movement and treatment system from a point of injury to a point of appropriate definitive care. Thus, the expeditionary facility is one link in a chain of care that includes first responder (self aid/buddy care, combat medics), forward resuscitative surgery, theater hospitalization for essential care within 12 hours of injury or illness, and evacuation out of theater for definitive care, tied together with en route care. The goal of expeditionary medical support is not to provide definitive care for patients in-theater until they can return to duty, it is to provide only enough care to stabilize patients sufficiently so that they can be evacuated out of the theater or otherwise placed in a disposition consistent with the theater commander's evacuation policies.[4]

A New Measure of Capability: The Medical STEP Rate

The goal of expeditionary medical support is to stabilize, triage and treat, and evacuate patients. First responders, expeditionary medical treatment facilities, and medical evacuation all contribute capabilities toward meeting this goal. They triage incoming patients, provide treatment to them if the level of care they can provide is sufficient, or stabilize them enough to enable them to be evacuated to a higher level of care. These capabilities, not the capacity to house patients, are what needs to be measured. Consequently, to measure the capacity of each component to provide its respective capabilities, we need to use not a static number, but a rate. We need to focus on the throughput of each stage, the rate at which that component of the system can evaluate, stabilize, triage and treat, and evacuate patients, or the *medical STEP rate*. The acronym captures the aspect of flow through a system, and the word "step" implies that each element provides an important step within a larger system.

Each component—first responders and CASEVAC, expeditionary medical treatment facilities, aeromedical evacuation, and definitive-care facilities—can be measured in terms of its medical STEP rate. The rate of an individual component depends on the resources available to it: The more ambulances, for instance, the higher the rate at which casualties can be transported from the point of injury to the expeditionary treatment facility; the more personnel and equipment at the expeditionary treatment facility, the more patients can be handled at a given time; the broader the specialized clinical capabilities at an expeditionary treatment facility, the broader the range of clinical interventions that can be rendered; and so on.

The system as a whole also has a medical STEP rate, which depends on the interaction between the components of the system. If

---

[4] *Expeditionary Medical Support (EMEDS)*, Air Force Tactics, Techniques, and Procedures 3-42.71 1, 2006.

aeromedical evacuation to definitive care is not available, patients will be forced to remain at the expeditionary medical facility. This creates a bottleneck, so that greater holding capacity and more caregivers will be needed to be able to provide care to new patients who arrive. The overall performance of the system can be optimized by ensuring that the interlayered component capabilities of EMEDS and aeromedical evacuation have matching medical STEP rates.

Using the STEP Rate Concept to Balance Capabilities and Requirements

Using the medical STEP rate as a measure of performance, the goal of a medical planner is to determine what resources are required in each element of the medical deployment system to achieve a desired medical STEP rate. The desired STEP rate, rather than the number of PAR, becomes the starting point. This determination of requirements encompasses both the types of resources (i.e., specific equipment and manpower) and the quantities of those resources.

The resources needed to achieve a desired medical STEP rate for a component such as EMEDS will largely depend on two factors: the patient influx to the facility and the medical STEP rate of any receiving component on the outflow side of the facility (e.g., aeromedical evacuation, local hospitals). Consider first the patient influx.

We saw above that the patient influx has two principal characteristics: the type and severity of patient conditions and the arrival rate. We also noted that the type and severity of conditions presenting may not be constant over time. For the purposes of assigning the appropriate resources to meet these requirements, only the patient conditions need to be specified. The STEP rate itself, not the resources to achieve a given STEP rate, will be adjusted to meet the needed rate. Planners will determine the resources to provide a given medical STEP rate, and logisticians will determine the STEP rate needed for a given deployment. This STEP rate depends dominantly on one aspect of the patient arrivals, the patient conditions.

The patient conditions in the three mission areas can differ quite widely. Most of the arrivals in the warfighter mission are relatively young, otherwise healthy individuals who have suffered trauma. In the

HUMRO and DSCA missions, the patients span a wider range of ages, are more balanced in numbers between the sexes, and often suffer from chronic health conditions. Indeed, the chronic health conditions may be what cause some patients to present.

The patient outflow consigns patients to some receiving element, such as the aeromedical evacuation system or, in the case of the DSCA mission, a local hospital. How well the STEP rates of the EMEDS and the receiving element match can affect the resources needed in the upstream facility. If the downstream receiving elements operate at a lower STEP rate for some period of time, the EMEDS unit may need additional holding capacity in order to maintain a given STEP rate. If the downstream elements have a higher STEP rate, the medical STEP rate for EMEDS will be completely specified by the patient conditions. Obviously, this is the desired state. But in some circumstances, especially where the aeromedical evacuation system is involved, the STEP rate may fluctuate with time due to battle conditions. The low points in these fluctuations may require that EMEDS units have the capacity to hold a certain number of patients to accommodate the inability of the aeromedical evacuation system to evacuate them.

These concepts are depicted schematically in Figure 3.1, using the analogy of water flow through buckets and pipes via pumps. In the figure, patients of a given condition arrive at some rate that may vary with time. The medical STEP rate of the deployed facility will determine the length of the queue of patients awaiting care or, more important, the *waiting time* until the patients receive appropriate care. After receiving care, most of these patients will be consigned to the outflow network, which may be another facility or the aeromedical evacuation system. The rate at which the outflow network can accept patients—its medical STEP rate—relative to that of the EMEDS will determine the backlog of patients that need to be held. These patients might be held at the EMEDS unit or at a Contingency Aeromedical Staging Facility (CASF). Therefore, given the rate of patient arrival, the desired maximum wait time for evaluation and provision of care, and the medical STEP rate of the outflow network, a required medical STEP rate and holding capacity can be calculated using queuing theory. The key elements are the linkage between the STEP rates, getting these rates to

Figure 3.1
Schematic Depiction of Medical STEP Rates and Related Capacities

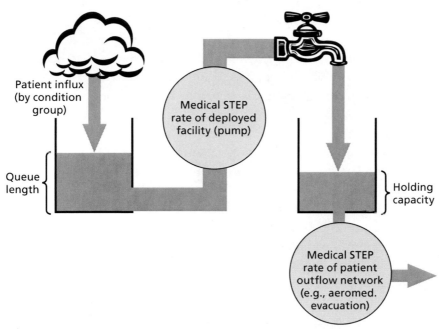

Patient influx
(by condition
group)

Medical STEP
rate of deployed
facility (pump)

Queue
length

Holding
capacity

Medical STEP
rate of patient
outflow network
(e.g., aeromed.
evacuation)

RAND *MG785-3.1*

match, and setting each to handle adequately the patient arrival rates
for each patient condition.

The queuing analysis should include the following details to cap-
ture the essential elements of the problem for determining the resource
types and levels needed to achieve a given medical STEP rate: a variety of patient arrival distributions beyond Poisson arrivals[5] for each ex-
amined patient condition; a queue discipline that reflects treatment of
patients in order of triage, not first-come, first-served; the maximum wait
time for patients to be treated (by condition type); the number of patients

_____

[5] A Poisson distribution models the number of independent events that occur in a fixed time
or space. A Poisson process is frequently used in queuing models and simulations because
many physical events tend to follow such a process. Many of the closed-form solutions for
queuing problems are based on Poisson arrival and departure. In the case of patient arrivals,
the assumption of identical, independent arrivals (key to a Poisson process) breaks down.

that can be treated simultaneously; and the distribution of the STEP rate of the downstream capability to which the patients are consigned.

Creating Unit Type Codes to Support Medical STEP Rates

Many possible patient conditions might be contemplated. In the mission of supporting the warfighter, a list of possible patient condition codes can be compiled, then, depending on simulations of battle, a list of expected frequencies of occurrence of each condition can be estimated. Resources needed to support these needs can then be determined in Task, Time, Treater File (TTTF) data. In this manner, resources needed to support a given number of PAR in a deployed, warfighting setting can be estimated. This is approximately the process currently used.

An additional challenge arises in the case of HUMROs and DSCA missions. The broad scope of these missions makes it impractical to attempt to estimate the expected frequency of all patient conditions. HUMRO deployments may be required even in the absence of a disaster. In the DSCA case, disasters can be of a wide range of types, including hurricanes, earthquakes, volcanic eruptions, floods, and the full spectrum of terrorist attacks, including attacks with chemical, biological, radiological, or nuclear weapons. Further, these incidents can occur in a wide range of populated areas.

As just one example, consider a large earthquake. In principle, an earthquake could occur in much of the United States, but it is most likely to occur somewhere along the San Andreas fault system in California or in the Cascadia zone in Oregon and Washington. If a major event occurred along the Hayward fault in Oakland, many of the hospitals might lose capability, because they are dominantly situated along the fault trace. In Los Angeles, on the other hand, the infrastructure is more dispersed, but the population is larger, and the spatial area of likely severe shaking is greater. Even if the time of day, the location of the focus, and the focal mechanism of an earthquake were known in advance, it would still be impossible to make a confident estimate of the resulting number and frequency of patient conditions. This uncertainty also holds for nearly every other disaster scenario.

Without an ability to predict with confidence the number and nature of patient conditions expected to present for the HUMRO and DSCA missions, it is desirable to have the force presentation be flexible enough to allow medical logisticians to assess rapidly the situation when it occurs and to express the requirements in terms that can be readily matched to existing UTCs. Hence, the goal is to establish resources in UTC packages that can be assembled rapidly to meet particular needs, rather than to try to predict the needs in advance and build UTC packages for them.

The medical STEP rate can serve this role, but the number of possible patient conditions needs to be reduced from potentially hundreds to a more manageable number. Further research could shed more light on the grouping choices, but one possibility would be to use the standard categories used in triage during any mass-casualty situation (i.e., urgent, immediate, delayed, minimal, and deceased (or expectant)).[6] It should be possible to estimate desired rates for these categories during HUMROs and DSCA events. If UTCs or combinations of modular UTCs existed for several medical STEP rates for each of these categories, defense coordinating officers would have an adequate vocabulary to relay the immediate needs, and the Air Force would have resources ready to meet them without deploying inappropriate resources.

Once medical STEP rates are determined for resources to meet some set of patient conditions, these resources need to be arranged in UTC capability units. The objective is to create the UTCs around medical STEP rate capabilities and to have them modular enough that they can provide any desired capability without deploying unneeded resources. The current EMEDS UTCs, while quite well constructed for the warfighter mission, do not fit the HUMRO or DSCA role as well. EMEDS emphasizes surgical capabilities—in equipment, supplies, and manpower—and some of these resources are in excess for some HUMRO and DSCA deployments. This excess delays the time to employment and increases the deployment footprint unnecessarily. Further, the current UTCs do not provide an ability to tailor a package that provides the right mix of infrastructure, equipment, man-

---

[6] Llewellyn, 1992.

power, and supplies to meet the full spectrum of pediatrics, geriatrics, OB/GYN, and other capabilities needed in HUMRO and DSCA deployments.

Exactly how to package resources into UTCs that meet these needs requires further study. For example, resources could be grouped into three categories: infrastructure and equipment, manpower, and sustainment. A lead infrastructure and equipment UTC might be created that provides some level of support that would be needed in virtually all deployments regardless of details of the patient conditions. This UTC might look quite similar to the current EMEDS Basic.[7] It could then be augmented by UTCs that provide additional capabilities, such as the ability to hold patients, intensive care unit (ICU) capability, surgical capability, and so forth. Each of these would be scaled according to the medical STEP rate.

The manpower UTCs could be similarly constructed and may or may not be joined with the infrastructure and equipment UTCs. Manpower UTCs could include a basic staffing team, general practices teams, surgical teams, pediatrics teams, geriatrics teams, psychiatric teams, and so forth.

Sustainment UTCs might include, for example, supplies and pharmaceuticals for surgery and general practice. This would enable provision of supplies such as insulin in instances like the Katrina relief effort. Again, all of these UTCs would be scaled to support a medical STEP rate for a given set of patient conditions. To meet a higher medical STEP rate, additional UTCs could be deployed.

Other factors come into play in UTC design. The analysis must take into consideration the distribution of manpower across the active duty, Air National Guard, and Air Force Reserves. From a management point of view, it is also desirable not to morcellate resources into a plethora of overspecialized UTCs. The goal should be a balance between the requirement that UTCs be modular enough to support

---

[7] A further policy decision concerns whether this UTC should contain its own expeditionary combat support. Such support is generally supplied by the Basic Expeditionary Airfield Resources UTCs and hence is not needed during the mission to support the warfighter. But these supporting UTCs are often not needed in HUMRO and DSCA deployments, and seeking such support can cost precious time and resources.

the full range of Air Force missions and the desire to minimize the overall number of distinct UTCs.

When all these considerations are taken into account, UTCs developed for STEP rates along modular lines would provide capabilities in terms of a dynamic measure of rates (not a static measure of beds); these capabilities would be matched among the various components of the deployable medical assets and would be flexible and agile in responding to the full range of missions. This construct would preserve and improve the already strong capabilities for support to the warfighter and could help shape improved capabilities for HUMRO and DSCA missions, for example, by restructuring the developing HUMRO Operational Capabilities Plan in terms of a medical STEP rate rather than the more traditional measure, beds.

CHAPTER FOUR

Summary and Conclusions

The key element for reshaping and measuring medical deployment capabilities is the proper choice of metric. We propose adopting the viewpoint of a medical STEP rate in defining, measuring, and presenting medical deployment capabilities. The STEP rate metric would reflect the process of stabilizing, triaging and treating, and evacuating patients. It departs from the more static measure, beds, and better captures the way deployed medical capabilities (i.e., EMEDS) operate—consisting of many elements in an interconnected system, EMEDS provides required medical care, moving patients to higher levels of care as needed.

We further propose that UTCs be defined around the concept of medical STEP rates and that various elements of the AFMS that support deployments attempt to match their medical STEP rates. We outlined a framework for designing medical deployment UTCs around medical STEP rates. To embrace the full flexibility of the STEP concept, the planning perspective needs to shift from contingency-based planning to adaptive planning. This would mean building modular UTCs for a given capability unit based on throughputs, rather than anticipating deployment requirements and building UTCs to meet them. The new, adaptive approach would give more flexibility during deployments and would allow a more tailored deployment to support HUMRO and DSCA missions, resulting in a smaller footprint for many deployments.

But identifying a metric and a construct to use that metric is not the same as devising an implementation plan. Challenges remain, and the best way to implement the change to a medical STEP rate metric of capability will require further research. How many medical STEP rates should be defined and around what criteria? These should be determined with all three deployment missions in mind. With the proper tools, resources required for given STEP rates can be determined for many patient conditions that span the mission areas of warfighting, HUMRO, and DSCA, but it would be impractical to develop UTCs for STEP rates for all possible patient conditions. Some grouping of conditions would be necessary, and analysis would be required to make sure that the various missions could be adequately supported. Even in light of these challenges, the approach seems promising for delivering a more agile, responsive, and capable medical deployment capability.

Current Air Force Medical Deployment Capabilities

The U.S. Air Force possesses two major medical deployment platforms: the Expeditionary Medical Support (EMEDS) system and the aeromedical evacuation system. These are both core competencies of the AFMS. This appendix briefly describes these missions and the resources that support them.

Expeditionary Medical Support

EMEDS is the Air Force system for providing essential medical care in forward locations. It consists of sets of tents, equipment, and personnel that can be built up in a modular fashion to provide increasing capabilities for larger numbers of patients. It is designed to provide primary care, dental care, and health protection to deployed personnel, as well as to stabilize casualties and prepare them for aeromedical evacuation.

The EMEDS modules are categorized by the number of inpatient beds they contain, but a more useful measure of EMEDS capability is the population at risk (PAR) that the units are intended to support. The system is designed so that as more personnel arrive at the deployed location, more tents, equipment, and medical personnel can be added to support the growing population.

The initial increment of medical capability is the Small Portable Expeditionary Aeromedical Rapid Response (SPEARR) team, which consists of 12 persons able to provide emergency surgical and critical care in a shelter of opportunity, using equipment carried in backpacks. An expanded version of SPEARR, which provides some additional equipment and a single tent, is intended to support a PAR of less than 500, typically during the phase when an airbase is being opened and established. The SPEARR team fits the definition of Level 2 (Casualty Collection and Forward Resuscitative Surgery) care.[1]

The next increment of capability is the EMEDS Basic, which builds upon the initial SPEARR team. It consists of three to four tents and has four patient beds intended for short-term holding only. EMEDS Basic is designed to provide medical support for a PAR of up to 2,000. It provides 24-hour sick call and emergency medical/dental care that includes medical command and control, preventive medicine, trauma resuscitation and stabilization, limited general and orthopedic surgery, critical care, primary care, dental care (including limited dental stabilization), aeromedical evacuation coordination, aerospace medicine, urgent care, and limited ancillary services.

EMEDS + 10 adds tents to EMEDS Basic, for a total of six or seven tents and 10 inpatient beds. It is intended to support a PAR of 2,000 to 3,000. EMEDS + 25 adds to EMEDS + 10, for a total of nine or 10 tents with 25 inpatient beds, to support a PAR of 3,000 to 5,000. The EMEDS + 25 beds provide complex medical/surgical inpatient capability, as well as personnel to support the medical wards. EMEDS + 25 provides the core infrastructure for specialty unit type codes (UTCs) (i.e., critical care, gynecology, otorhinolaryngology, neurosurgery, oral surgery, ophthalmology, thoracic/vascular surgery, urology, mental health triage, and combat stress management). Additional subspecialty surgical UTCs can also be added at the Air Force Theater Hospital (AFTH) level to include neurosurgery, oral surgery, thoracic/vascular surgery, ophthalmology, otolaryngology, urology, gynecology, and head and neck surgical team, which when combined with previous increments can support a PAR of 5,000 to 6,500.

Each of the EMEDS configurations deploys with enough supplies for seven days of operation. EMEDS Basic is not considered to have

---

[1] *Health Services*, Air Force Doctrine Document 2-4.2, 2002, Appendix, p. 75, defines the complete set of levels of medical care.

inpatient beds; its four beds are intended for short-term holding (i.e., less than 24 hours). Aeromedical evacuation is assumed to be necessary and available. Even though the larger EMEDS + 10 and + 25 configurations do have inpatient beds and critical care capability, they are also not intended to provide patients with long-term care. Patients are still expected to be evacuated out of the theater for definitive care, reconstructive surgery, and rehabilitation.

While the SPEARR team can deploy and function in austere conditions, the EMEDS configurations from Basic on up are dependent on expeditionary combat support. EMEDS brings tents and climate-control units, but with the exception of a generator carried by SPEARR, it is reliant on expeditionary combat support to provide electricity to power its systems, including the medical equipment. In addition, EMEDS requires water, ice, fuel, waste disposal, and communications, as well as billeting for its personnel.[2]

Aeromedical Evacuation

Aeromedical evacuation[3] is an enduring capability of the AFMS, with roots tracing back to World War II. The aeromedical evacuation mission is to move patients supervised by medical personnel via fixed-wing aircraft to higher levels of medical care. The aeromedical evacuation system frequently serves as a conduit between deployed capabilities such as EMEDS (and the Army-equivalent combat support hospital) and higher levels of medical care such as Landstuhl Regional Medical Center in Germany and Walter Reed Army Medical Center in Mary-

---

[2] Additional information on EMEDS can be found in *Expeditionary Medical Support (EMEDS)*, Air Force Tactics, Techniques, and Procedures 3-42.71, 2006, and *Health Services*, Air Force Doctrine Document 2-4.2, 2002.

[3] Aeromedical evacuation is distinct from two related patient-movement missions, CASEVAC and MEDEVAC. Casualty evacuation (CASEVAC) is a general term used mainly by services other than the Air Force to refer to unregulated casualty movement aboard any vehicle or aircraft. Medical evacuation (MEDEVAC) generally refers to movement of casualties accompanied by medical attendants via rotary-wing aircraft within the theater.

land. A large majority of the aeromedical evacuation assets lie outside the active duty forces, within the Air Reserve component.

Aeromedical evacuation forces are modular and can build from a small liaison team to a full Theater Aeromedical Evacuation System (TAES). Aeromedical evacuation elements provide command, control, communications, patient care, and system support. Much like EMEDS, aeromedical evacuation resources are packaged based on a modular, building-block principle. The major components of the aeromedical evacuation system are staging facilities and manpower teams, described below.

The Mobile Aeromedical Staging Facility (MASF) is a 15-person, communications-capable UTC that provides supportive/resuscitative nursing care for patients awaiting airlift. The MASF can manage a patient throughput of 40 to 60 patients in a 24-hour period. It is designed to provide forward support with the smallest footprint and is usually located at or near an airfield.

The Contingency Aeromedical Staging Facility (CASF) is an expeditionary platform that consists of one of the ground components necessary for patient movement. It is intended for airlift hubs that receive and transport a large number of patients. The CASF can serve as an extension of the EMEDS/AFTH and provides patient reception, complex medical/surgical nursing care, and limited emergent intervention. CASF personnel ensure that patients are medically and administratively prepared for flights.

CASFs are built in modular increments from three personnel UTCs that are combined in various numbers to form aeromedical staging facilities of 25-, 50-, 100-, and 250-bed configurations. CASF capability includes operating a staging facility for continuous (24-hour/7-days-per-week) operations. Critically ill patients awaiting airlift are generally cared for at either the nearest medical facility with the required capability (e.g., the EMEDS/AFTH) or on a short-term basis (not to exceed 72 hours) by Critical Care Air Transport Teams (CCATTs) at the CASF location for patients awaiting airlift.

The aeromedical evacuation crew is a five-person UTC comprising two flight nurses and three aeromedical evacuation technicians.

The aeromedical evacuation crew provides in-flight nursing care for up to 10 stabilized patients per crew member.

A CCATT is a three-person team that enhances the ability of the aeromedical evacuation system to transport critically ill patients. Each CCATT comprises one intensive-care or non-intensive-care physician (depending on the patient care needs), one critical-care nurse, and one cardiopulmonary craftsman who is specially trained to provide critical care/specialty care during transport. The CCATT is added to the basic aeromedical evacuation crew to offer a higher level of care to stabilized patients during aeromedical evacuation staging and flight when this higher level of clinical capability is required. The CCATT has been referred to as the "flying ICU" team. The theater validating flight surgeon in the Patient Movement Requirements Center coordinates with the sending physician to determine when a CCATT is required.

For DSCA operations, the Air Force aeromedical evacuation system can support patient evacuation accomplished through the National Disaster Medical System (NDMS). The U.S. Transportation Command validates the requirement to support civilian authorities. Once validated, the Air Mobility Command/Tanker Airlift Control Center (AMC/TACC) is the lead operational authority for aeromedical evacuation planning, coordinating, and, when directed, executing DSCA support under the National Response Framework[4] in the United States.[5]

Current Capabilities and CONOPS

The AFMS provides a tiered approach to flowing tailored medical capabilities in response to a mission requirement. The AFMS's doctrinal framework is to provide essential medical capability with the first deployment of personnel, to build and sustain an appropriate level of

---

[4] *National Response Framework*, 2008.

[5] Additional information on aeromedical evacuation can be found in *Aeromedical Evacuation (AE)*, Air Force Tactics, Techniques, and Procedures 3-42.5, 2003, and *Health Services*, Air Force Doctrine Document 2-4.2, 2002.

capability throughout an operation's phases (deployment, employment, and redeployment), and to ensure that an appropriate level of care exists while at-risk personnel are present. Key contextual factors in determining the appropriate level of medical capabilities include, but are not limited to, the threat scenario, expected casualty rates, expected casualty types, potential disease and non-battle injuries (DNBI), the theater commander's evacuation policy, evacuation distance, evacuation time frames and potential delays, airlift availability, and the PAR.

The PAR is generally defined in terms of military personnel supported by the medical capability (on today's battlefield, it may include government civilians, coalition partners, and, in some cases, contractors). A significant distinction can be drawn between a PAR under a combat deployment scenario (i.e., medical requirements for a population in some defined contact with enemy forces, with resultant planning based on estimated categories and volumes of combat injuries as well as DNBI rates) and a PAR within a DCSA operation (i.e., where a DSCA may have medical scope only to support responders or medical scope to provide care to the general population of civilians affected by the disaster, including the potential for traumatic injury post-disaster and, very likely, acute community health care requirements in the population at large).

When creating and sizing UTCs, medical planners build to the appropriate level based on PAR, expected combat wounds, evacuation policy, evacuation delay, and evacuation distance, to name a few of the most significant factors. PAR is dominant, and the resources needed to support a given PAR depend on the expected frequencies and types of medical conditions in a given population. Not only do these populations differ significantly over the three missions the AFMS is called upon to support, other fundamental characteristics of these environments also differ in ways that impact planning and programming.

Bibliography

Aeromedical Evacuation (AE), Air Force Tactics, Techniques, and Procedures 3-42.5, 1 November 2003.

Bowman, Steve, Lawrence Kapp, and Amy Belasco, *Hurricane Katrina: DoD Disaster Response*, CRS Report for Congress, Washington, D.C.: Congressional Research Service, 19 September 2005.

Davis, Lynn E., Jill Rough, Gary Cecchine, Agnes Gereben Schaefer, and Laurinda L. Zeman, *Hurricane Katrina: Lessons for Army Planning and Operations*, Santa Monica, Calif.: RAND Corporation, MG-603-A, 2007.

Dorland, Peter, and James S. Nanney, *Dust Off: Army Aeromedical Evacuation in Vietnam*, Washington, D.C.: Center of Military History, United States Army, 1982. As of September 1, 2008:
history.amedd.army.mil/booksdocs/vietnam/dustoff/

Expeditionary Medical Support (EMEDS), Air Force Tactics, Techniques, and Procedures 3-42.71, 27 July 2006.

Franco, Crystal, Eric Toner, Richard Waldhorn, Beth Maldin, Tara O'Toole, and Thomas V. Inglesby, "Systemic Collapse: Medical Care in the Aftermath of Hurricane Katrina," *Biosecurity and Bioterrorism: Biodefense Strategy, Practice, and Science*, Vol. 4, 2006, pp. 135–146.

Gabriel, Richard A., and Karen S. Metz, *A History of Military Medicine, Volume 2: From the Renaissance Through Modern Times*, New York: Greenwood Press, 1992.

Greenwood, John T., and F. Clifton Berry, Jr., *Medics at War: Military Medicine from Colonial Times to the 21st Century*, Annapolis, Md.: Naval Institute Press, 2005.

Health Services, Air Force Doctrine Document 2-4.2, 11 December 2002.

Lister, Sarah A., *Hurricane Katrina: The Public Health and Medical Response*, CRS Report for Congress, Washington, D.C.: Congressional Research Service, 21 September 2005.

Llewellyn, Craig H., "Triage: In Austere Environments and Echeloned Medical Systems," *World Journal of Surgery*, Vol. 16, 1992, pp. 904–909.

Moseley, T. Michael, *Air Force Support to Hurricane Katrina/Rita Relief Operations: Successes and Challenges*, Washington D.C.: Office of the Chief of Staff of the U.S. Air Force, August–September 2005.

Nanney, James S., *The Air Force Medical Service in the Persian Gulf War*, Bolling AFB, Washington, D.C.: United States Air Force, Office of the Surgeon General, 1992.

———, *The Air Force Medical Service and the Persian Gulf War: A Ten-Year Retrospective*, Bolling AFB, Washington, D.C.: United States Air Force, Office of the Surgeon General, n.d.

National Response Framework, Washington, D.C.: Department of Homeland Security, January 2008. As of September 1, 2008: http://www.fema.gov/emergency/nrf/

Office of the Air Force Surgeon General. As of September 1, 2008: http://www.sg.af.mil/history/index.asp

Pomeroy, G. W., "Dividends from OEF, OIF Pay Off for Medics in Katrina Aftermath," *Air Force Print News Today*, 30 September 2005. As of September 1, 2008: http://www.af.mil/news/story_print.asp?storyID=123011988

Scott, William B., David A. Fulghum, and Craig Covault, "The Second Storm," *Aviation Week and Space Technology*, 12 September 2005, pp. 20–22.

Townsend, Frances Fragos, *The Federal Response to Hurricane Katrina: Lessons Learned*, Washington D.C.: The White House, February 2006.